The ED Blueprint

Steps to Restoring Sexual Health and Confidence

Adesoji Abe

TABLE OF CONTENTS

CHAPTER 1. INTRODUCTION TO ERECTILE DYSFUNCTION

Erectile dysfunction (ED) affects millions of men worldwide. This condition is defined as the inability to achieve or maintain an erection sufficient for satisfactory sexual performance. ED can be a warning sign of underlying health issues, such as cardiovascular disease, diabetes, or hormonal imbalances. It can also be triggered by psychological factors like stress, anxiety, or depression.

In this booklet, we'll explore both natural and scientific remedies that can help you regain control of your sexual health. Whether you're dealing with occasional erectile difficulties or more persistent challenges, this guide will equip you with knowledge, tips, and strategies to manage and improve ED naturally.

1. Understanding the Causes of Erectile Dysfunction

Before diving into remedies, it's crucial to understand the causes of ED. While aging increases the likelihood of ED, it is not an inevitable part of getting older. Common causes include:

Physical Causes:

- **Cardiovascular Diseases:** Conditions like atherosclerosis (hardening of the arteries) restrict blood flow to the penis, making it difficult to achieve an erection.

- **Diabetes:** High blood sugar levels can damage blood vessels and nerves involved in sexual response.

- **Obesity:** Excess weight contributes to hormonal imbalances and reduced circulation.

- **Hormonal Issues:** Low testosterone, thyroid problems, or prolactin imbalances can lead to reduced sexual desire and performance.

- **Medications:** Drugs for high blood pressure, depression, and other conditions can have side effects that impact erectile function.

Psychological Causes:

- **Stress and Anxiety:** Psychological stress can interfere with your brain's ability to send the necessary signals to trigger an erection.

- **Depression:** ED can be both a symptom and a consequence of depression.

- **Relationship Issues:** Lack of intimacy or communication with a partner can also contribute to ED.

2. Exploring Natural Remedies for Erectile Dysfunction

While modern medicine offers effective treatments like PDE5 inhibitors (e.g., Viagra), many men prefer natural alternatives that address the root causes of ED. Here, we'll explore scientifically backed natural remedies that can complement your health regimen.

a. Herbal Treatments:

i. Panax Ginseng (Korean Red Ginseng)

- **How it works:** Known as the "herbal Viagra," Panax ginseng enhances nitric oxide production, which relaxes the blood vessels in the penis and promotes blood flow. Studies suggest it may improve erection strength and duration.

- **Dosage and Use:** A typical dosage is 600-1000 mg, taken three times a day.

- **Scientific backing:** A 2002 study found that 60% of men taking Panax ginseng noticed improvement in their symptoms.

- **Precautions:** Avoid use if you have uncontrolled hypertension.

ii. L-Arginine

- **How it works:** L-Arginine is an amino acid that helps make nitric oxide, which is critical for erections because it helps blood vessels relax. This improves blood flow to the penis.

- **Dosage:** Studies recommend 5 grams per day, but some men may benefit from lower doses (2-3 grams).

- **Research evidence:** A 1999 study found that men with organic ED who took L-arginine saw significant improvements in sexual function.

- **Safety:** Can cause low blood pressure in high doses, so check with your doctor if you're on any medication.

iii. Yohimbine

- **How it works:** Extracted from the bark of the African Yohimbe tree, Yohimbine increases blood flow to the penis by blocking certain neurotransmitters and increasing nitric oxide.

- **Dosage:** 5-10 mg, taken three times per day.

- **Studies:** Clinical trials have shown that Yohimbine is effective in treating mild to moderate ED, especially when psychological causes are involved.

- **Side effects:** Anxiety, increased heart rate, and dizziness.

iv. Ashwagandha (Indian Ginseng)

- **How it works:** Traditionally used in Ayurvedic medicine, Ashwagandha helps reduce cortisol levels and improves sexual function by boosting energy levels and reducing stress.

- **Dosage:** 300-500 mg, twice daily.

- **Research:** Studies show Ashwagandha enhances sexual performance, particularly in men with stress-induced ED.

b. Diet and Nutrition:

i. Omega-3 Fatty Acids

- **Source:** Found in fish like salmon, flaxseeds, and walnuts.

- **How it helps:** Omega-3s improve heart health by reducing inflammation and increasing blood flow, which directly impacts erectile function.

- **Tip:** Add fish oil supplements or consume fatty fish twice a week to promote better circulation.

ii. Antioxidant-Rich Foods

- **Source:** Berries, dark chocolate, spinach.

- **How it helps:** Antioxidants reduce oxidative stress, which can damage blood vessels and affect sexual health.

- **Tip:** Eat a variety of colourful fruits and vegetables daily to support overall sexual health.

c. Zinc-Rich Foods

- **Source:** Oysters, pumpkin seeds, spinach.

- **How it helps:** Zinc is essential for testosterone production, which is critical for sexual desire and performance.

- **Tip:** Aim for foods rich in zinc or consider a supplement if your levels are low.

d. Lifestyle Changes:

i. Quit Smoking

- Smoking damages blood vessels, making it harder to maintain an erection. Quitting can dramatically improve erectile function.

- **Tips for Quitting:** Use nicotine replacement therapies (patches, gums), counselling, or mobile apps to track progress.

ii. Moderate Alcohol Consumption

- Alcohol depresses the central nervous system, making it harder to get and maintain an erection.

- **Tip:** Limit intake to 1-2 drinks per day or avoid it altogether for better results.

iii. Regular Physical Activity

- Exercise improves cardiovascular health, which is crucial for erectile function. Activities like running, swimming, or cycling can enhance blood flow and stamina.

- **Tip:** Aim for at least 30 minutes of moderate exercise, 5 times a week.

e. Physical Exercises to Improve Erectile Health:

i. Kegel Exercises

- **How to do them:** Contract the pelvic floor muscles as if you're trying to stop urinating, hold for 5 seconds, then release. Repeat 10-15 times, three times daily.

- **Benefit:** Strengthens the muscles responsible for erectile function, helping to maintain an erection for longer.

ii. Aerobic Exercises

- Aerobic exercises like jogging, swimming, or even brisk walking can improve cardiovascular health and ensure better blood flow to the penis.

- **Tip:** Incorporate daily aerobic exercises to enhance overall health and sexual function.

f. Psychological Factors and Stress Management

Stress, anxiety, and depression are major contributors to ED. Addressing mental health can lead to significant improvements in sexual function.

i. Mindfulness Meditation:

- Meditation helps calm the mind and reduces performance anxiety. It also improves self-awareness, which can alleviate stress linked to sexual performance.

- **Tip:** Practice deep breathing and mindfulness meditation for 10-15 minutes each day to reduce stress levels.

ii. Cognitive Behavioural Therapy (CBT):

- Therapy can help men overcome negative thoughts and anxiety related to sexual performance. CBT has been shown to improve ED in men whose dysfunction is tied to psychological factors.

- **Tip:** Seek a professional therapist specializing in sexual health or anxiety disorders.

g. Communication with Partners:

- Open communication with a partner can reduce pressure, improve intimacy, and alleviate ED. Discuss fears, desires, and ways to support one another.

4. Medical Treatments: When Natural Remedies Aren't Enough

Sometimes, lifestyle changes and natural remedies may not provide sufficient results. In these cases, medical treatments may be necessary:

PDE5 Inhibitors (e.g., Viagra, Cialis): These medications increase blood flow to the penis, making it easier to achieve and maintain an erection.

- **How they work:** They block the enzyme that causes the penis to lose its erection.

- **Usage:** Take the pill 30-60 minutes before sexual activity.

- **Side effects:** Headaches, flushing, dizziness, and nasal congestion.

Vacuum Erection Devices (VED): These mechanical pumps help create an erection by drawing blood into the penis. A constriction ring is placed at the base to maintain the erection.

Penile Injections: Medication like alprostadil can be injected directly into the penis to stimulate an erection.

Surgery: In severe cases, penile implants may be considered.

5. Case Studies: Success Stories and Real-World Applications

Include real-world stories of individuals who have successfully improved ED through natural remedies, lifestyle changes, and medical intervention. Each case study should detail their challenges, the remedies they tried, and their eventual success, adding personal credibility to the guide.

Frequently Asked Questions (FAQ)

- **Can I combine natural remedies with prescription medications?**

- Yes, but consult with a doctor first to avoid potential interactions.

- **How long do natural remedies take to work?**

  - Some remedies, like L-arginine, may show results in a few weeks, while others, like lifestyle changes, take longer.

- **What's the safest treatment for ED?**

  - The safest treatment is dependent on the underlying cause, and consulting a doctor is recommended before beginning any new treatment.

Chapter 2. Exploring Natural Remedies for Erectile Dysfunction: Practical Guide to Preparation

1. Panax Ginseng (Korean Red Ginseng)

Ingredients:

- 600-1000 mg Panax ginseng extract (available in capsule or powder form)

- Water (if taking the powder form)

Preparation Steps:

i. **Purchase high-quality Panax ginseng extract** from a reputable health store or online retailer. Ensure it's marked as "standardized" for consistent potency.

ii. **For capsules**: Simply take the recommended dosage (600-1000 mg), usually 1-2 capsules, three times a day with meals. Always follow the manufacturer's dosage instructions.

iii. **For powder form**: Mix 1 teaspoon (equivalent to 600-1000 mg) of Panax ginseng powder into a glass of warm water, stir well, and drink. You can also mix the powder into a smoothie, tea, or juice for better taste.

iv. **Usage Tip**: Take Panax ginseng for a minimum of 4 weeks to start noticing improvements in erectile function. It's best used as a long-term supplement to improve blood circulation and energy.

v. **Precautions**: Avoid taking Panax ginseng if you have uncontrolled high blood pressure. It's also best to avoid caffeine when using this remedy, as both are stimulants.

---

2. L-Arginine

Ingredients:

- L-Arginine powder or capsules (500 mg or 1000 mg per dose)
- Water (if using powder)

Preparation Steps:

i. **Purchase L-Arginine powder or capsules** from a trusted health supplement store. Make sure it's labelled as pure L-Arginine without additives.

ii. **For capsules**: Take 2-5 grams (2000-5000 mg) per day, divided into two doses. For example, take one 1000 mg capsule twice a day, preferably before meals. Follow the dosage recommended on the packaging.

iii. **For powder form**: Mix 1-2 teaspoons (2000-5000 mg) of L-Arginine powder in a glass of water, stir until dissolved, and drink once in the morning and once in the evening.

iv. **Usage Tip**: Use L-Arginine consistently for at least 2-3 weeks before evaluating its effectiveness. Combining it with an exercise regimen can enhance its blood-flow-boosting effects.

v. **Precautions**: Avoid taking too much L-Arginine in one dose, as it can cause gastrointestinal discomfort or low blood pressure in high amounts.

3. Yohimbine

Ingredients:

- Yohimbine supplements (usually available in 5 mg tablets)

Preparation Steps:

i. **Purchase Yohimbine supplements** from a reliable source. Look for supplements that clearly state the dosage on the label (usually 5-10 mg).

ii. Take 5 mg of Yohimbine once in the morning and once in the evening, with meals to avoid stomach upset. Start with the lowest dose and increase if tolerated.

iii. **Usage Tip**: Use Yohimbine for at least 2-4 weeks to start noticing improvements. It works best for individuals experiencing ED due to psychological stress or anxiety.

iv. **Precautions**: Yohimbine can cause anxiety, increased heart rate, and high blood pressure in sensitive individuals. Start with a small dose and monitor your body's response. Consult your doctor before use, especially if you have any heart conditions.

---

4. Ashwagandha (Indian Ginseng)

Ingredients:

- Ashwagandha root powder or capsules (300-500 mg per dose)
- Water (if using powder)

Preparation Steps:

i. **Purchase Ashwagandha supplements** from a reliable health store, ensuring the product is organic and free from harmful additives.

ii. **For capsules**: Take one 300-500 mg capsule twice daily with meals. Follow the recommended dosage on the packaging.

iii. **For powder form**: Mix 1 teaspoon of Ashwagandha root powder into warm water or milk. Stir thoroughly and drink twice a day (morning and evening).

iv. **Usage Tip**: Take Ashwagandha consistently for at least 6-8 weeks to see results, especially in reducing stress-related ED and improving overall vitality.

v.   **Precautions**: Ashwagandha is generally safe, but if you have thyroid issues or are on medication for autoimmune diseases, consult your doctor before use.

5. Dietary Changes: How to Prepare Erectile-Boosting Meals

Diet plays a crucial role in supporting erectile function. Here's how to easily incorporate ED-friendly ingredients into your daily meals.

a. Omega-3 Fatty Acids (from Fish like Salmon)

Ingredients:

- Fresh salmon fillet (about 200-300 grams per serving)
- Olive oil (1 tablespoon)
- Lemon juice (1 tablespoon)
- Fresh herbs (dill or parsley for flavour)

Preparation Steps:

i. **Preheat the oven** to 200°C (400°F).

ii. **Drizzle the salmon fillet** with olive oil and lemon juice, and season with fresh herbs, salt, and pepper.

iii. **Place the salmon on a baking sheet** lined with parchment paper and bake for 12-15 minutes, or until the fish flakes easily with a fork.

iv. **Serve with** steamed vegetables or a green salad for a heart-healthy, erection-boosting meal.

v. **Tip:** Include salmon or other fatty fish in your diet 2-3 times per week to boost cardiovascular health and improve erectile function.

b. Antioxidant-Rich Smoothie

Ingredients:

- 1 cup mixed berries (blueberries, strawberries, raspberries)

- 1 handful spinach

- 1 tablespoon chia seeds

- 1 cup unsweetened almond milk

- 1 tablespoon honey (optional)

Preparation Steps:

i. **Place all the ingredients** in a blender.

ii. **Blend until smooth**. Add more almond milk if needed for desired consistency.

iii. **Drink this smoothie** every morning to support overall sexual health. The antioxidants in the berries help reduce oxidative stress and improve blood flow.

iv. **Tip**: Make this smoothie part of your daily routine for long-term benefits. You can switch up the fruits for variety.

c. Zinc-Rich Snack (Pumpkin Seeds Trail Mix)

Ingredients:

- 1 cup roasted pumpkin seeds (pepitas)
- ½ cup almonds
- ½ cup sunflower seeds
- ½ cup dried cranberries

Preparation Steps:

i. **Mix all ingredients** in a large bowl.

ii. Store the trail mix in an airtight container and eat ¼ cup as a snack once or twice a day. The high zinc content in pumpkin seeds supports testosterone production and sexual health.

iii. **Tip:** Take this snack on the go for a quick and nutritious boost to your day.

d. Physical Exercises: Step-by-Step Instructions

Incorporating specific exercises into your daily routine can further enhance your sexual health.

1. Kegel Exercises for Men

Step-by-Step Instructions:

i. **Identify your pelvic floor muscles** by trying to stop urinating mid-stream. The muscles you contract to do this are the pelvic floor muscles.

ii. **Once identified**, contract these muscles for 5 seconds, then relax for 5 seconds.

iii. **Repeat 10-15 times**, three times a day. You can do Kegels lying down, sitting, or standing.

iv. **Tip**: Perform these exercises consistently to strengthen your pelvic floor muscles and improve erectile function. You should start noticing improvements in 4-6 weeks.

---

2. Aerobic Exercise: How to Start a Routine

Step-by-Step Instructions:

i. **Start with a 5-10 minute warm-up** (brisk walking, gentle stretching).

ii. **Choose an aerobic activity** such as jogging, swimming, or cycling.

iii. **Perform the activity** for 30-45 minutes, at least 5 times a week.

iv. **Cool down** with a 5–10-minute walk or stretching session.

v. **Tip**: If you're new to exercise, start slowly and gradually increase your intensity. Aerobic exercises improve cardiovascular health, which is essential for erectile function.

e. Additional Natural Remedies for Erectile Dysfunction: Detailed Preparation Guide

1. Maca Root (Lepidium meyenii)

Ingredients:

- Maca root powder or capsules (500 mg – 1500 mg per dose)
- Water or milk (if using powder)

Preparation Steps:

i. **Purchase organic Maca root powder** or capsules from a trusted source. Look for products that are specifically labelled for ED or energy enhancement.

ii. **For capsules**: Take 500-1500 mg of Maca root daily. Start with 500 mg once a day and gradually increase based on how your body responds. Always follow the manufacturer's instructions.

iii. **For powder form**: Mix 1 teaspoon of Maca root powder into a glass of warm water, milk, or your favourite smoothie. Stir well until dissolved.

iv. **Usage Tip**: Maca root can help boost libido and stamina over time. Use it consistently for at least 4-6 weeks to notice the benefits.

v. **Precautions**: Maca root is generally safe, but if you have a hormone-sensitive condition, consult with your doctor before use.

2. Horny Goat Weed (Epimedium)

Ingredients:

- Horny goat weed extract (500 mg – 1000 mg per dose)

Preparation Steps:

i. **Purchase horny goat weed supplements** from a reliable source. Look for a product standardized for icariin, the active compound.

ii. **For capsules**: Take 500-1000 mg daily with meals. Start with a smaller dose and assess how your body reacts before increasing the dosage.

iii. **Usage Tip**: Horny goat weed works best when taken regularly. Use it for at least 4-8 weeks for noticeable improvements in erectile function.

iv. **Precautions**: Some individuals may experience mild side effects such as dizziness or rapid heartbeat. Reduce dosage if necessary and consult a doctor if the side effects persist.

3. Tribulus Terrestris

Ingredients:

- Tribulus terrestris extract (500 mg per dose)

Preparation Steps:

i. **Purchase Tribulus terrestris supplements** from a reliable health store. Ensure it contains a standardized percentage of saponins (the active compound).

ii. **For capsules**: Take 500 mg of Tribulus terrestris extract daily. Some products may recommend dividing the dosage, so follow the packaging instructions.

iii. **Usage Tip**: This herb helps increase testosterone levels and improve sexual function, especially in men with low testosterone. Use it consistently for 4-6 weeks for best results.

iv. **Precautions**: Tribulus terrestris is generally safe, but excessive use may cause stomach upset. Stick to the recommended dose and consult a healthcare provider if you have any underlying health conditions.

4. Pomegranate Juice

Ingredients:

- 1 cup fresh pomegranate juice (or store-bought 100% pure pomegranate juice)

Preparation Steps:

i. **Buy fresh pomegranates** or 100% pure pomegranate juice from a grocery store.

ii. **For fresh juice**: Cut the pomegranate in half and use a juicer to extract the juice from the seeds. Pour it into a glass.

iii. **For store-bought juice**: Make sure it's unsweetened and pure. Drink 1 cup daily.

iv. **Usage Tip**: Pomegranate juice is rich in antioxidants that improve blood flow and reduce oxidative stress, both of which can help with ED. Drink it regularly for at least a month to see its benefits.

v. **Precautions**: Avoid drinking pomegranate juice if you are on blood-thinning medications, as it may interfere with the medication.

5. Ginkgo Biloba

Ingredients:

- Ginkgo Biloba extract (120 mg per dose)

Preparation Steps:

i. **Purchase Ginkgo Biloba extract** from a health food store. Look for supplements with a standardized concentration of 24% flavone glycosides and 6% terpene lactones.

ii. **For capsules**: Take 120 mg once a day with a meal. It is best taken in the morning as it can be mildly stimulating.

iii. **Usage Tip**: Ginkgo Biloba improves blood flow, particularly to the genital area, which can help men experiencing ED due to poor circulation. Take it consistently for 4-6 weeks.

iv. **Precautions**: If you are on blood thinners or have a bleeding disorder, consult your doctor before taking Ginkgo Biloba.

6. Watermelon (Citrulline)

Ingredients:

- Fresh watermelon (1 cup)

- Lemon juice (optional)

Preparation Steps:

i. **Cut fresh watermelon** into small cubes and place them in a blender.

ii. **Blend the watermelon** until smooth. You can add a splash of lemon juice for extra flavour.

iii. **Drink 1-2 cups daily**, especially before engaging in sexual activity. Watermelon contains citrulline, an amino acid that helps relax blood vessels and improve blood flow, similar to how Viagra works.

iv. **Usage Tip**: While not as potent as prescription ED medications, regular consumption of watermelon can help improve erection quality over time.

v. **Precautions**: Watermelon is generally safe, but if you have a medical condition that limits your intake of high-water fruits, consult your doctor.

7. Fenugreek

Ingredients:

- Fenugreek seeds (1 tablespoon)

- Water (1 cup)

Preparation Steps:

i. **Soak 1 tablespoon of fenugreek seeds** in a cup of water overnight.

ii. **In the morning, strain the seeds** and drink the water on an empty stomach. This method is believed to improve sexual stamina and boost libido over time.

iii. **Usage Tip**: You can also purchase fenugreek supplements and follow the dosage on the packaging (usually 500-600 mg daily). Fenugreek is particularly effective for improving testosterone levels.

iv. **Precautions**: Avoid fenugreek if you are allergic to legumes or on blood-thinning medications.

By breaking down the steps for each remedy and including easy-to-follow instructions, this booklet will serve as a practical guide for anyone looking to naturally improve their erectile health. It makes the process approachable and simple, even for those who may be unfamiliar with herbal supplements, diet changes, or exercise routines.

f. Lifestyle and Mind-Body Therapies for Erectile Dysfunction

1. Acupuncture

What to Do:

i. **Find a licensed acupuncturist** who specializes in sexual health or treating ED.

ii. **Schedule a series of sessions**, usually once a week, for 6-12 weeks.

iii. **Usage Tip**: Acupuncture can help alleviate psychological causes of ED, such as anxiety and stress, by promoting relaxation and energy flow throughout the body.

iv. **Precautions**: Ensure that the acupuncturist follows proper hygiene practices and uses sterile needles.

2. Pelvic Floor Physical Therapy

What to Do:

i. **Consult a pelvic floor physical therapist** who can teach you specific exercises to strengthen your pelvic muscles.

ii. **Follow a customized exercise regimen** that targets the muscles used for erection and ejaculation. This can include variations of Kegel exercises and other pelvic muscle toning routines.

iii. **Usage Tip**: Regular therapy can result in significant improvements in erectile function, especially for those experiencing ED due to weak pelvic muscles or surgery recovery.

3. Comprehensive Lifestyle Adjustments for Erectile Dysfunction

Nutrition and Diet

- **Low-fat Diet**: Emphasize the importance of a heart-healthy, low-fat diet. Foods rich in omega-3 fatty acids (like salmon, flaxseeds, and walnuts), whole grains, and leafy greens help improve circulation and reduce the risk of ED.

- **Avoid Excessive Sugar and Processed Foods**: Explain how these can cause inflammation, disrupt blood flow, and negatively affect sexual function.

- **Probiotic-rich Foods**: Include options like yogurt and fermented vegetables that boost gut health, which is connected to overall well-being, including sexual health.

Exercise

- **Aerobic Exercise**: Encourage readers to incorporate at least 30 minutes of aerobic exercise daily, such as walking, cycling, swimming, or jogging. These activities improve cardiovascular health, which directly impacts erectile function.

- **Strength Training**: Explain the benefits of strength training to improve testosterone levels, reduce body fat, and enhance libido. Include exercises such as squats, lunges, and push-ups.

Stress Reduction Techniques

- **Mindfulness Meditation**: Describe how practicing mindfulness can help reduce performance anxiety and promote relaxation, leading to improved sexual function. Provide a simple, step-by-step meditation guide that users can easily follow.

- **Yoga for Sexual Health**: List some yoga poses (such as bridge pose, cobra, and pelvic lifts) that improve blood flow to the pelvic region, reduce stress, and increase flexibility, which can help with sexual performance.

g. Holistic and Alternative Therapies for Erectile Dysfunction

Massage Therapy

- **Pelvic Massage**: Discuss how massaging the pelvic area can help increase circulation and alleviate tension in the muscles that support sexual function.

- **Full-body Massage**: Explain the importance of relaxation and stress relief in improving ED symptoms. Recommend professional or self-massage techniques, such as Swedish massage, to promote overall well-being.

Herbal Infusions and Teas

- **Herbal Tea Recipes**: Provide easy-to-follow recipes for teas that can support sexual health, such as:

  - **Ginseng Tea**: Known for boosting stamina and energy levels.

  - **Ashwagandha Tea**: Helps reduce stress and improve sexual function.

  - **Damiana Tea**: A natural aphrodisiac that enhances sexual desire and improves mood.

Example Recipe:

  - **Ingredients**: 1 teaspoon of dried ginseng root, 1 cup of water.

  - **Instructions**: Boil water, add ginseng root, and let it steep for 10 minutes. Strain and enjoy.

h. Psychological and Emotional Support for Erectile Dysfunction

Counselling and Therapy

- **Sex Therapy**: Explain how working with a certified sex therapist can help men and their partners address the emotional and psychological factors contributing to ED.

- **Cognitive Behavioural Therapy (CBT)**: Provide a brief overview of CBT and how it can help men reframe negative thoughts about sexual performance.

Communication with a Partner

- **Open Conversations**: Include a section on how to have open and supportive conversations with a partner about ED. This can help reduce performance pressure and create an understanding atmosphere.

- **Couples' Exercises**: Offer ideas for intimacy-building exercises that focus on non-sexual affection, such as cuddling, kissing, and massages, to build emotional connection without pressure.

i. Daily Routine Planner for Erectile Health

Provide a practical, sample daily routine to help readers incorporate these remedies and lifestyle changes into their day-to-day lives. Include:

- Morning: Fenugreek water + 10 minutes of pelvic exercises.

- Mid-day: A walk or 30 minutes of aerobic exercise.

- Afternoon: Herbal tea (such as ginseng) + mindfulness meditation.

- Evening: Healthy dinner (high in leafy greens and omega-3 fatty acids).

- Before bed: Maca root supplement + a few minutes of relaxation exercises or yoga.

j. Final Thoughts: A Motivational Message

Erectile dysfunction can feel overwhelming, but remember, you are not alone in this journey. Millions of men around the world face the same challenges, and many have successfully regained their confidence and vitality through persistence, lifestyle changes, and natural remedies.

The path to better sexual health is not about quick fixes—it's about making gradual improvements in how you live, nourish your body, and care for your mind. Every small step count, whether it's adding a new herb to your routine, practicing daily exercises, or simply taking time to reduce stress.

Believe in your ability to overcome this. Your body and mind have a remarkable capacity to heal and adapt, and by following the guidance in this booklet, you're already on the right track. Be patient with yourself and stay consistent, and over time, you'll start seeing positive changes—not only in your sexual health but in your overall well-being.

Remember, true strength lies in taking charge of your health. By taking these steps today, you're moving towards a more confident, vibrant version of yourself. Keep going, stay committed, and know that a fulfilling, healthy, and happy life is within your reach. You deserve it.

19. Frequently Asked Questions (FAQ)

Include a FAQ section to address common questions such as:

- "How long will it take before I see results?"

- "Can I use multiple remedies at once?"

- "Are there any side effects of these herbs?"

- "Do I need to consult a doctor before using these remedies?"